# HAVE YOUR CAKE...
# AND EAT IT TOO!

Donald Gorbach

ISBN-10 1978434952
ISBN-13 978- 1978434950

"DON'T SAVE ANYTHING FOR A SPECIAL OCCASION.
BEING ALIVE IS THE SPECIAL OCCASION."

—ANONYMOUS

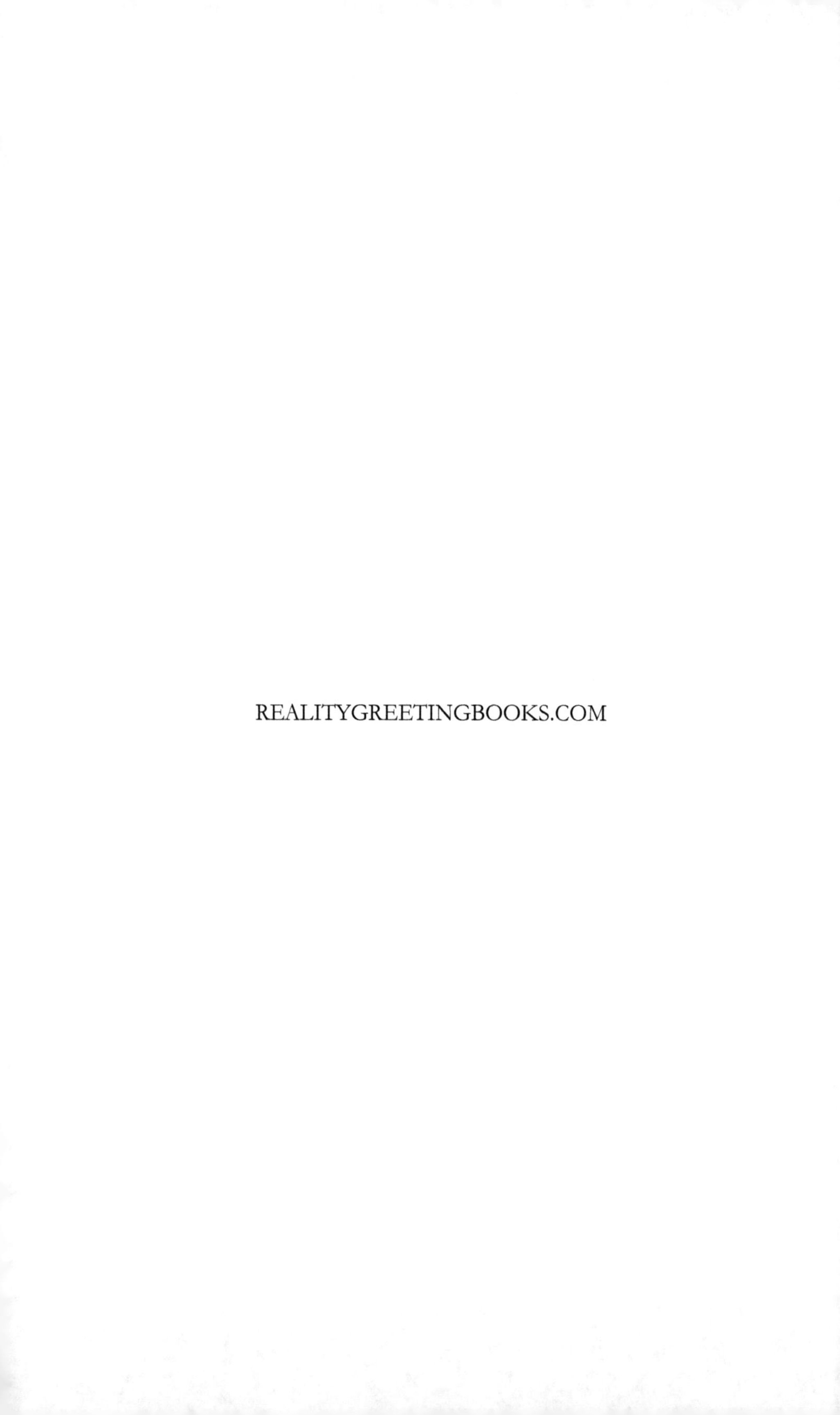

REALITYGREETINGBOOKS.COM